Project Time Travel

A Beginner's Guide to Physical Eternal Life

By:

Paeti Gustav Xaviers

This book is dedicated to all humanity,
with love and all due and appropriate respect.

Project Time Travel is an application of the principles found in the Theory of Life Perpetuity - Theory of Physical Eternal Life - published under the penname of Paeti Gustav Xaviers.

Time Travel should be approached under the care of a physician.

I. Introduction:

Perpetuity is the secret to existence. It is the secret to energy. It is the secret to life. A Perpetuity is something that once set in motion, would continue in motion forever, with no additional energy required to maintain it. In order to set a perpetuity in motion, it must be ignited. Impregnation is the ignition of a perpetuity. The perpetuity ignited when a human being is conceived it the perpetuity of the energy of his life: his lifetime. Doesn't it follow that if lifetime (one's life energy) is perpetual, the body it is a part of should be able to live forever? In fact, it is possible.

Along with his lifetime, the human being has basically three components: physical body, mind and spirit. Of these components, two must be nurtured: physical body and spirit. The mind is the go between and the regulator of the living energy.

Let's discuss the time through which a human being must live.

Time is an existence of the 4th dimension that exists within the three physical dimensions. It must be passed through. It is like there is perpetually 4th dimension barriers that physical beings must pass through, and survive the passage, in order to exist or live for any period of time.

Whether or not a living being physically transforms (evolves) or dies at any point in time depends on how smoothly the being passes through these time barriers. If the being passes through the barrier, it transforms and continues. It further matures or ages. It lives another day. The more consistently smooth a being matures, transforms and continues determines the length of time the being will live.

What causes physical death is trauma caused by erratic or chaotic transformations or continuances as the being passes through the time barriers (passes through time). The body of the being reaches the point where it is unable to withstand any more trauma, it hits a barrier and literally gets its lights knocked out (it dies). A human being must master the proper way to time travel.

Well, if life energy within a human body is eternal (a perpetuity), why do human beings die? One only be familiar with the Genesis of the Holy Bible to figure out how mankind got started on his death oriented path. Believe it or not, the answer is all too obvious. Eve ate an apple. From that point on, it was pretty much doomsday for man.

II.

Human life and the beings it is composed of are Holy. The energy that gives the life to the human being is Divine. The three components of a human being, the spirit, mind and body, have the ability to also become Divine. Once all of the components of a human being become Divine, and along with the Divinity of the human being's life energy, the human being becomes one complete Divinity with Eternal Physical Life. Something Divine is something that is a perpetual energy within itself.

The physical order in which a human being achieves Divinity is first, mind. The mind nurtures the spirit and the human being must nurture his/her own body. So, how does the mind become Divine?

The mind becomes Divine when it achieves a state of being completely righteous. Sinfulness within the mind is totally absent. The mind becomes righteous, or sinful, based upon a human being's thoughts and actions. To achieve Divinity most rapidly, one must constantly and continuously think and behave in a righteous manner.

What is righteousness? Righteousness is making the conscious decisions of choosing God over Earth, but at the same time being equally respectful of both. As the human being then makes decisions and behaves accordingly, the mind becomes more and more righteous.

The mind is not a physical component of the human being upon birth. It becomes manifested, as it could ever possibly be, upon the Holy union between the mind, spirit and body. When this marriage takes place it makes the complete human being Divine.

Next in line is the human spirit. Upon birth, the human spirit is not physical and is shrouded in death. It can only conquer death by becoming physical. In order to become physical, spiritual matter must be produced. The way spiritual matter is produced is by the spirit being nurtured by the righteousness of the mind. Spiritual matter is the composition of a human being's soul and is physical matter in another dimension.

Last in line is the human body. It is the component, of all of human components, that is most vulnerable to death. It must be nurtured to pass as smoothly and efficiently through the 4th dimensional time barriers that exist within the three physical dimensions as possible. It must pass through the barriers with as little trauma as it is able. In order to do this, it must be nurtured by the human being himself/herself in such a manner that this effect takes place.

The human body is a temple. You can read about this in the book of Corinthians in the Holy Bible. It is the temple of the spirit. The temple has an altar. The altar is the human being's mouth. Whatever a human being consumes is worship of, an offering to or a sacrifice to God. The highest order ritual of worship is the burnt offering. This ritual being performed must only be done in the most proper and respectful manner. In order to become Divine, a human being must make burnt offerings at some point in time.

Everything else consumed is a sacrifice of some sort, unless the consumption is of a liquid. Consuming liquid is the most proper and respectful way to nourish the body. It is the most righteous – not sacrificing anything. Human beings have no right to sacrifice anything of Earth in order that they live themselves.

Until such time as the human being is blessed with Physical Divinity, burnt offerings should be made with the left hand (the "God" hand). Sacrifices should be made with the right hand (the "humble" hand). The process of nurturing the body should also be done with the right hand. A human being should not engage in the ritual of burnt offerings until physical maturity has been reached. Caution should be used when deciding the type of sacrifice. A sacrifice is any physical food the human being eats. More about burnt offerings will be discussed later.

III.

In order to time travel most properly and efficiently, the physical body must process the energy of its lifetime in an efficient manner. To do this, the body systems, which process the energy, must be kept in sync with the lifetime energy. There should be a smooth flow, or volley, of energy that that causes the body to pass through the time barriers at the same rate, or as near the same rate as possible, as the lifetime energy itself.

Physical matter, the body, moves more slowly than the human being's mind and spirit. This is why it must be nurtured appropriately. If the body is moving too slowly or too quickly, it becomes ill – to the maximum of becoming cancerous, which is a degeneration of the physical body, or dying of a heart attack. If it starts moving too slowly or too quickly, the balance of the flow of energy between lifetime and the body fluctuate, and action must be taken to encourage the energy flow to be back in sync. If not balanced, health issues most often occur.

So the human body must be nourished, preferably by consuming only liquids, in order to pass through time most in tune with the energy of the being's lifetime. First, let's talk in general about the way the body functions.

The human body is a masterpiece. It is in God's image. It is fully capable of achieving physical life eternal on its own, provided it is properly and sufficiently nourished – and not to forget righteous. So what nourishment does the body absolutely require?

First and foremost, the body needs minerals. Minerals are necessary for the smooth functioning of the body's internal organs. The organs that process the lifetime energy. All of the minerals required, when consumed in conjunction with other required nutrients, is found in the composition of water. The consumption of water not only provides the necessary minerals, it promotes digestive health.

Water need not only be consumed in conjunction with other nutrition. It is perfectly righteous to consume water alone. If not enough water is consumed, the body becomes dehydrated due to shortage of minerals. If your lips are dry, that is the signal from your natural self that you need minerals from water.

After nourishing the internal organs and minding the health of the digestive system through the consumption of water, bone and muscle health are the most critical. Bone health is promoted by consuming calcium. Muscle health is promoted by the consumption of protein. All of the necessary vitamins for healthy time travel are naturally produced by a well nourished and efficiently running human body. If a human body is healthy, it need not consume vitamins from an outside source.

III. Nutritionalization:

I call the process of nurturing the body "nutritionalization." The body should be nutritionalized immediately upon waking from sleep, or as soon thereafter as possible. Nutritionalization is the first action that should be taken when a human being awakes. Thereafter, at any particular time of day, the body should only be nutritionalized when necessary so as not to cause an overload of nutrition. The sign that nutritionalization is necessary is when the body starts to feel really hungry or the stomach growls. That is the signal that the body has completed the process of completely digesting its prior consumed nutritionalization and it is time for more nourishment.

The consumption process should also be done with a smooth flow. The body should not be shocked, or traumatized, with sudden bursts of nutrition. One should also take their time, not rush through the consumption of the liquid nourishment by gulping the sequence of liquids. It may be consumed a bit quickly than just slowly sipping, but not by gulping. (Roughly, it should take 10 to 20 minutes to completely consume a glass of nutrition, takeing up to 3 sips at a time.) Gulping down the nutrition would overload the digestive system and slow the body enough that it will get out of sync with the energy of lifetime.

Start nutritionalizing with a 16oz. glass of water. This should be unfiltered water. Tap water. You want the minerals of the Earth, in whatever state the Earth is currently in. Tap water should be fine in most cases, unless the water is incredibly polluted. The body will naturally absorb the minerals and reject the chemicals that may be present.

Following water, drink an 8oz glass of whole milk, which is the nutrition of calcium and a little protein. The milk should be followed by a shot of protein. A shot of protein can be prepared from a powder of whey protein, preferably mixed with water. Then you have to work your way out of the buildup to or climax of the nutritionalization. You need an anticlimax to make the nutrition flow. Accomplish this in the same way the nutrition was approached, only backwards: after the shot of protein, drink another 8oz glass of whole milk, which will be followed by another 16oz glass of water.

Now, let's briefly discuss situations of pollution or the intake of liquids that contain other than minerals, calcium and protein.

There will always be times when somethings other that the necessary minerals, calcium and protein are consumed. Of course, God knew the Earth could be polluted by man. This other stuff that is consumed could be additives that cause the nutrition to taste better. The body naturally knows what it needs and will naturally discard anything and everything it does not need. The discard is eliminated from the body via a bowel movement. Urine is a composite of mostly water that the body has an excess of or is finished processing. Note that urine is also a natural cleanser for the genitals, and should not be forced to dry quickly with anything such as toilet paper. Most properly, you should "drip dry." Toilet paper should only be used to wipe the anal area when a bowel movement is made.

Consumption of anything into the body (the temple) by way of the mouth (the alter) causes a fluctuation in the energy flow from lifetime to the body. It is the body's natural immune system that protects the body from becoming ill as a result of the fluctuation. Think of the immune system as a rubber band. When there is a fluctuation, the immune system will stretch, and upon completion of the consumption it will begin to move back to its original, healthy shape. By the time the consumption is completely digested, the immune system should be returned to its original condition if the body is healthy and was nutritionalized properly.

Extreme fluctuations in energy flow stresses the immune system. For a period of time, the immune system will be strong enough to return itself eventually to its best health. However, continuous extreme stretching, or stressing, of the immune system could cause it to become permanently out of shape to the point where one more fluctuation could cause it to break. Realizing this, if an individual immediately changes his "sacrifice consumption" lifestyle to proper and healthy nutritionalization (proper worship), the immune system could eventually heal and return to a strong healthy state. However, depending upon the seriousness of the damage, the immune system may never heal.

Consumption into the body (temple) by way of the mouth (alter) is a manner or ritual of worship.

Everyday nutritionalization constitutes everyday worship: a manner. It is like saying a prayer. When physical food is consumed, it is a sacrifice: a ritual. Consumption of substances that increase the speed of the energy of lifetime is considered a burnt offering: a ritual of the most power.

Physical food should only be consumed in the event of an emergency. Typically, an emergency is called if, during the digestion process, the individual feels lightheaded or passes out. At that point, the individual should consume physical calories, but they should be empty calories that provide as little energy as possible. For example, I typically eat potato chips. Then the individual should lie down and rest, or try to sleep, in order that the mind tend to balancing the energy flow as quickly as possible without interference. By lying down, the entire body will be concentrated on bringing the body back into sync with the lifetime energy. It is recommended that a prayer be said or thought either before or after the rest.

The body does not need to consume calories to burn for energy. It is energized naturally by the energy of lifetime. It is the consumption of calories that causes the energy flow to fluctuate and stress the immune system. The objective for greater health is to consume as few calories as possible without sacrificing nutrition. The purpose of nutritionalizing the body is so that the body processes are healthy enough to process the lifetime energy, not to create a counter-energy.

IV.

Here are some signals that your body is moving too slowly or not working efficiently:

ALWAYS TIRED OR FALLING ASLEEP
(when not your normal rest periods) – This is your signal that your body is moving to a near extreme of slowness. Your entire being needs to concentrate in order to bring the energy flow back in sync, without interruption or interference. The body needs to catch up to your lifetime energy.

PROTRUDING STOMACH – This is a signal that you are under-nourished. You are suffering from some degree of malnutrition. You are consuming a lot of garbage and not the proper nutrients in the proper way (the process of nutritionalization).

EXCESS BODY FAT/OBESITY – This signals that your body is not processing your lifetime energy efficiently. As a result, it is moving too slow. The lifetime energy that passed to the body is being stored instead of being used. Typically, excess body fat is coincident with malnutrition.

AGING APPEARANCE – This is the signal that as the body is passing through the time barriers, it is crashing, causing trauma. The body is not easily and efficiently passing through time.

ILLNESS – Anything from a common cold to cancer – or heart attack.

Here are some signals that your body is moving too quickly:

DIZZINESS/PASSING OUT – You should consume empty calories to slow your body down and then lie down so your being and process the calories and adjust your energy flow.

UNDERWEIGHT/LACK OF SUFFICIENT BODY FAT – You should nutritionalize more often, perhaps even when your stomach is not growling or you are not feeling really hungry. Just upon feeling the emptiness of the stomach. But not too much nutrition should be consumed at one time (don't nutritionalize and nutritionalize again as soon as you are finished). Wait a little bit of time inbetween. Give your body a chance to digest the nutrition before consuming again. Wait to feel what signals your body sends you.

ILLNESS – Anything from a common cold to cancer – or heart attack.

V.

Treatment for a body too slow or too fast:

A body that is out of sync with its lifetime energy should be treated, or continuance at the out of sync pace could cause illness – possibly severe. Running too slow is the most common. If your body is running too slow, it can be "revved up." Caffeine is the natural substance to use to accomplish this. But do NOT consume caffeine while nutritionalizing. Consume it in between nutritionalizations. Caffeine consumption causes the body to start and run the processing of lifetime energy, including stimulating the immune system which is part of the processing of lifetime energy.

If you are going to drink coffee or tea, drink it black – no sugar or milk. Not drinking it black is the same thing as consuming caffeine while nutritionalizing. Highly caffeinated diet soft drinks are good. But make sure the soft drinks are zero calories. Don't worry about the chemicals the soda may contain. The body will naturally reject them, causing an eventual bowel movement. Nutrilization slows the body down. You do not want to stimulate the body processes (slow the body down) by consuming calories. You want to rev the processes up.

Caffeine is also a natural cure for illnesses – from the common cold to cancer. It stimulates the immune system, a body process. When ill, consuming caffeine in between periods of nutritionalization re-encourages the immune system to get moving and get back in shape.

If your body is running too fast, you better slow down if you want to keep your health. DON'T DO STRENUOUS EXERCISE…this speeds the body up in drastic bursts. It causes extreme trauma as you body is trying the pass through time. You want your body to flow through time…you want your energy flow to be smooth –

not high/low, high/low, low/high, with a drastic changes from one point in time to the next.

Notes:

Don't rush. If your body is too slow or too fast, it needs to heal. You've probably been living a death oriented lifestyle for a long time. The longer living that lifestyle, the more healing that needs to be done. The healing process takes time and should be done naturally. Don't consume pills or inject anything (medications/nutritions) into the body. That causes the body shock and trauma. It's a BURST, not a natural flow. Don't cause your body energy levels to become erratic, by not nutritionalizing when necessary or by doing physical exercise.

Time moves at an extremely fast pace and you want to flow with it, not keep crashing into the time barriers. You want to flow through the time barriers. Constant crashing causes eventual death.

And don't get upset about a possible negative affect on your appearance. When your body is healthy and the energy is flowing and being processed efficiently, you will literally transform. It could appear as if time has been reversed. You will become your perfect body weight and turn into the most physically beautiful self of your being. But it takes time.

VI.

I mentioned that making a burnt offering is the
ritual with the most power. Proper substances to
use to make a burnt offering are tobacco or
marijuana. These substances are smoked. During
the process of smoking, God is literally
summoned. But heed my word, prior to
attempting a burnt offering, you had best be sure
your mind is filled with righteously sincere
thoughts, not just seeking physical pleasure or
having a good time, or serious health issues could
result. It is considered an act of blasphemy and
your temple could be damned. That is why so
many people become ill or die as a result of
smoking.

SMOKING CIGARETTES

Smoking a cigarette is like calling God on the

telephone. You could have a problem that you would like some input on, or you might just want to have a casual chat like with a friend. Smoking stimulates the mind and opens your thoughts to God. He can read them. He receives them. It is the next step up from praying. When the smoke is exhaled, your thoughts are sent to God (you are participating in the conversation).

There is a proper way to smoke a cigarette.

First, you must smoke with your left hand. Think of your left hand as your "God" hand. Second, you must open your mouth and chant while you are inhaling and exhaling the smoke. After dragging some smoke into your mouth, open your mouth (the wider is the more causal – widest is the most pleasurable) and whisper/pronounce "mah." For the most part, the smoke will wrap around your tongue, not be drawn into the lungs. When you exhale, whisper/pronounce "who."

If you are frightened or nervous about calling God on the phone, relax your body and mind by sipping on a beer while you are smoking. Practice makes perfect. Don't get drunk. The absolute maximum should be four beers. Don't drive or be partying. You should smoke outside and, for best results, be alone.

Work up to a casual phone call. As you practice opening your thoughts and sending them to God, if it's a problem you were struggling with you will start to realize that you are inspired about it – suddenly you can figure it out. God eventually will answer you. It could be immediate, if He picks up the phone. Or you could be on "call waiting." Sometimes you will find your resolve while you sleep or sometimes the answer will just pop into your head at an odd point in time. But if you used proper respect when you placed your call and used the proper manner, God will get back to you...if He doesn't, then it is something God wants you to figure out for yourself. God is not the book of knowledge that you can continuously look things up in quickly. God wants you to use your mind and think.

SMOKING MARIJUANA

By smoking marijuana you are not just stimulating your mind and opening your thoughts to God…you are opening your ENTIRE MIND to God whenever you are "high." You are making a personal visit to His house and knocking on the front door, not just calling Him on the phone. Watch your step.

The difference in the proper way to smoke marijuana as compared to smoking common tobacco is that it should be done with your right hand (your "humble" hand) and the smoke should be dragged into the lungs as directly and deeply as possible. Then the smoke should be held in the lungs until the lungs feel as if they are going to burst. No chanting is necessary with marijuana. It is recommended that you be in a suitable environment, as well: dim lights (perhaps a candle) and you are alone without anyone else who could interrupt you. Soft music is also nice.

Caution: Do NOT drink beer or other alcoholic beverages in combination with smoking marijuana. You could lose complete control over you mind and you will find yourself in a totally obliterated mental state. When that happens, God has cut you off. Marijuana abuse could entice God to take your mental abilities away – you could become permanently mentally ill.

DO NOT consume alcohol in any form other than beer or use narcotics or drugs other than marijuana. God will slam His door in your face. With continued abuse, God could take away your ability to think acutely, or it could cause coma or death.

VII.

Once you realize the absolute Holiness of existence, adjust your manner and behave accordingly, you will start to become more comfortable with God. When that happens, you are at the point where you can experiment with time traveling for fun.

It is possible to really time travel, pushing your body, spirit, mind and soul through time barriers of the 4th dimension faster than the rate of other people. How fast depends on the health and efficiency of your body, and, of course, your righteousness. This causes a physical reaction and could make things happen – either for you personally or for the entirety of mankind.

Time travel for fun is extremely easy, but should be approached with caution. Holiness, remember? All you have to do is during some interval between acts of nurtitionalization, consume caffeine while smoking cigarettes. The reaction will take place when you go to sleep (when you are unconscious) and something will happen. Something will happen to you, around you, or it may be something you will see on the news. But your time travel triggered a reaction – like a nuclear chain reaction – but relative to time, not matter.